THE SHIATSU HANDBOOK

Stress-Relieving And Health-Promoting Techniques And Strategies

FRANK JACKSON

Contents

CHAPTER ONE
An Introductory

Shiatsu is a Japanese bodywork technique that entails applying pressure to specific points on the body to promote healing, relaxation, and general well-being.

The Japanese term "shiatsu" translates to "finger pressure," which is the primary technique utilized in this modality. Shiatsu is founded on the principles of traditional Chinese medicine and combines acupuncture, acupressure, and massage techniques.

Shiatsu practitioners believe that vital energy, known as Qi (pronounced "chee"), circulates through a network of meridians or energy channels in the body. The body is healthful when the flow of Qi is balanced and harmonious.

Nevertheless, when the flow of Qi is obstructed or disrupted, it can result in physical or emotional discomfort, pain, or illness. Shiatsu seeks to restore the body's Qi balance and promote natural healing.

The recipient remains completely clothed and reclines on a

comfortable mat or futon during a typical shiatsu session.

Concentrating on specific points along the meridians or energy pathways, the practitioner applies pressure and manipulates the recipient's body using their fingertips, palms, elbows, and knees. Shiatsu may also involve massages, joint rotations, and other techniques for relieving stress, enhancing circulation, and promoting relaxation.

Shiatsu is renowned for its holistic approach, which considers the recipient's physical, emotional, and energetic aspects.

It is frequently used to alleviate stress, reduce muscle tension, relieve discomfort, enhance sleep, and improve overall health. Shiatsu is also utilized as a complementary treatment for a variety of health conditions, including digestive issues, respiratory issues, hormonal imbalances, and musculoskeletal disorders.

Importantly, shiatsu should only be performed by a trained and certified practitioner who is familiar with the principles and techniques of this modality.

As with any form of bodywork, it is essential to discuss any health concerns, discomfort, or preferences with the practitioner during the session. Shiatsu is generally safe for the majority of individuals, but it may not be appropriate for everyone, particularly those with certain medical conditions or who are pregnant.

Before attempting shiatsu or any other form of complementary therapy, it is always advised to consult with a healthcare professional.

Philosophy And Principles Of Shiatsu

Shiatsu is guided by a number of fundamental principles and philosophies. These principles, which are rooted in traditional Chinese medicine (TCM) and Japanese philosophy, serve as the basis for the shiatsu approach and techniques. Among the fundamental principles and philosophies of shiatsu are the following:

• Qi (Ki): In shiatsu, Qi, also known as Ki in Japanese, is the central concept. It refers to the vital energy that travels through the body along channels or meridians. The smooth passage of Qi is necessary for maintaining health and wellbeing, and imbalances or blockages in Qi can result in discomfort, pain, or illness.

Shiatsu seeks to balance and harmonize the body's Qi flow, thereby enhancing its natural healing capacities.

• Yin and Yang: Shiatsu acknowledges the complementary and opposing forces in the universe represented by Yin and Yang. Yin is associated with darkness, repose, and cooling, whereas Yang is associated with light, activity, and heat.

In shiatsu, the practitioner attempts to balance the Yin and Yang energies within the body in order to promote health and harmony.

• Meridians and Acupoints: Shiatsu is based on the concept of meridians or energy channels, which are believed to be pathways through which the body's Qi travels. These meridians correspond to particular organs, systems, and bodily functions.

Along these meridians are specific locations known as acupoints or tsubos in Japanese, where the Qi can be accessed and manipulated to restore equilibrium. Shiatsu practitioners utilize acupressure techniques to apply pressure and stimulate these acupoints in order to release blockages, tension, and facilitate the free passage of Qi.

• Shiatsu takes a holistic approach to health and well-being, acknowledging that the body, mind, and spirit are interconnected and mutually influence one another.

Shiatsu practitioners consider the emotional, mental, and energetic aspects of the recipient in addition to the physical symptoms. Shiatsu's purpose is to restore balance and harmony to the entire person, fostering a sense of wholeness and well-being.

• Shiatsu practitioners approach their clients with unconditional positive regard, which entails a nonjudgmental, receptive, and compassionate disposition. This allows the client to unwind, release tension, and be open to the healing process in a safe and supportive environment.

• Ki Diagnosis: Shiatsu practitioners frequently employ a form of energetic diagnosis known as "Ki diagnosis" to evaluate the client's condition and determine the most effective treatment.

This may involve palpation, observation, and intuition in order to discern imbalances in the client's Qi and determine areas of concentration for the session.

• Self-Care and Empowerment: Shiatsu emphasizes self-care and encourages the recipient to take an active role in their health and well-being. Shiatsu practitioners may suggest self-care practices, such as stretching, breathing exercises, lifestyle modifications, and dietary changes, to promote the client's ongoing health and wellness.

These are some of the fundamental shiatsu principles and philosophies. It is essential to note that different shiatsu styles and schools may have their own techniques and approaches, but they generally adhere to these fundamental principles.

CHAPTER TWO
Shiatsu's Health And Well-Being Advantages

Shiatsu provides numerous health and well-being benefits. As a form of holistic bodywork, shiatsu addresses not only the physical but also the emotional, mental, and energetic aspects of a person, thereby promoting overall balance and harmony. Among the principal benefits of shiatsu are:

• Shiatsu is renowned for its profoundly relaxing and stress-relieving effects on the body and psyche. During a shiatsu session, the pressure and manipulations serve to release tension and stress, promoting relaxation and calming the nervous system.

This can reduce the physical and mental effects of stress, including muscle tension, anxiety, and fatigue, leaving the recipient feeling more relaxed, revitalized, and centered.

• Shiatsu can alleviate a variety of painful conditions, including muscular tension, joint rigidity, and chronic pain. During a shiatsu session, the applied pressure and stretches can help loosen tense muscles, improve circulation, and stimulate the body's natural pain-relieving mechanisms.

Shiatsu is beneficial for conditions such as back pain, neck pain, migraines, arthritis, and fibromyalgia, according to reports.

• Shiatsu seeks to balance and harmonize the flow of Qi or vital energy throughout the body. Shiatsu can restore vitality, increase energy levels, and promote a sense of well-being by relieving blockages and enhancing the circulation of Qi. This can be especially beneficial for those who feel exhausted, depleted, or drained of energy.

• Shiatsu encourages the recipient to develop a greater awareness of their body, its sensations, and its requirements. Through the application of pressure, stretches, and manipulations, the recipient can develop a more intimate relationship with their body, thereby enhancing body awareness and mindfulness.

This increased body awareness can lead to improved self-care practices, better posture, and a deeper comprehension of one's physical and energetic state.

• Shiatsu's calming effects can also enhance the quality of your sleep. Shiatsu can induce a state of relaxation that can contribute to improved sleep by reducing stress and tension. Numerous shiatsu patients report enhanced sleep, including deeper, more restful sleep and fewer sleep disturbances.

• The connection between the body and emotions is acknowledged by shiatsu. Emotional well-being can be improved through the discharge of tension and the balancing of Qi. Shiatsu can reduce anxiety, depression, and emotional stress symptoms, leaving the recipient feeling more balanced, centered, and emotionally resilient.

• Shiatsu's capacity to promote relaxation, reduce stress, and enhance circulation can have a beneficial effect on the immune system. Reducing stress and relaxing can support a healthy immune response, which can contribute to an improvement in overall health and wellbeing.

• Shiatsu promotes self-care and empowers recipients to take an active role in their health and well-being. Shiatsu can support personal development, empowerment, and a deeper understanding of one's own body, mind, and emotions through increased body awareness, self-reflection, and self-care practices.

It is essential to note that shiatsu is not a replacement for medical care, and it is always recommended to consult a qualified healthcare professional with any health concerns.

As a complementary therapy, shiatsu can provide numerous health and well-being benefits, including relaxation, pain alleviation, enhanced energy flow, emotional well-being, and personal development.

Understanding The Meridians And Acupressure Points: The Body's Energy Channels

Traditional Chinese medicine (TCM) and shiatsu rely heavily on meridians and acupressure points.

They are believed to be the channels and points through which Qi or Chi, also known as vital energy, circulates throughout the body. Fundamental to the practice of shiatsu is knowledge of meridians and acupressure locations.

Meridians are channels or pathways through which Qi circulates in the body. In TCM, there are twelve major meridians that correspond to specific organs or bodily functions, such as the lung meridian, heart meridian, spleen meridian, etc.

Each meridian corresponds to a specific organ or system and has its own distinct pathway. It is believed that these meridians are interconnected and constitute a network that facilitates the circulation of Qi throughout the body. It is believed that the meridians are responsible for nourishing the body's organs, muscles, tissues, and other structures, as well as sustaining the body's overall balance and harmony.

Acupressure Points: Also known as acupoints or tsubos in Japanese, acupressure points are specific points along the meridians where Qi can be accessed and influenced. Each acupressure point along the meridians has its own distinct characteristics and functions. By applying pressure, stretching, or other techniques to acupressure points, the flow of Qi can be controlled, stimulated, or slowed. Typically, these sites are located in specific anatomical locations, such as depressions, indentations, or hypersensitive areas.

In shiatsu, practitioners apply pressure, stretches, and other techniques to stimulate or sedate acupressure points along the meridians using their hands, fingertips, palms, elbows, or other body parts. By manipulating these points and meridians, shiatsu seeks to regulate the flow of Qi, release blockages, and restore the energy system's balance and harmony.

Shiatsu's comprehension of meridians and acupressure points is based on the principles of TCM, which views the body as an interconnected network of energy channels and stresses the importance of maintaining a harmonious flow of Qi for optimal health and well-being.

It is important to note, however, that the concepts of meridians and acupressure points are based on theories of traditional Chinese medicine and may not be recognized in the same manner by other medical systems or Western scientific standards.

Nonetheless, many shiatsu practitioners and recipients find the concepts of meridians and acupressure points beneficial for comprehending and manipulating the body's energy system during shiatsu sessions.

CHAPTER THREE
The Healing Balance Of Yin And Yang

Yin and Yang are fundamental concepts in both traditional Chinese medicine and Chinese philosophy, including shiatsu.

They are believed to be present in all aspects of the universe, including the human body, despite being opposing forces. The concept of Yin and Yang is used to characterize the dynamic and interdependent nature of the universe, as well as the necessity of maintaining a balance between these opposing forces for optimal health and well-being.

Yin represents the passive, receptive, and feminine qualities, whereas Yang represents the active, assertive, and masculine qualities.

Yin and Yang are frequently depicted as a circle with a swirl of black and white, symbolizing the interplay between light and darkness, heat and chill, expansion and contraction, and other contrasting qualities. Additionally, the circle represents the continuity and cyclical nature of these opposing forces.

Health is attained when Yin and Yang are in a state of harmonious equilibrium within the body. Any disturbance or imbalance between these forces can lead to illness, distress, or pain.

Consequently, the purpose of shiatsu is to restore or maintain the balance between Yin and Yang in the body in order to promote health and healing.

Shiatsu practitioners use a variety of techniques, including pressure, stretches, and other manipulations, to stimulate or sedate specific acupressure points along the meridians in order to regulate the passage of Qi and restore Yin and Yang balance.

For instance, if a patient exhibits symptoms of excess Yang energy, such as heat or agitation, the shiatsu practitioner may employ techniques to subdue or pacify the Yang energy and promote Yin energy.

If a person has excess Yin energy, such as numbness or lethargy, the shiatsu practitioner may employ techniques to stimulate or invigorate the Yang energy in order to restore balance.

The goal of balancing Yin and Yang is not to eliminate one force in favor of the other, but rather to achieve a state of equilibrium between them. It is essential to note that the balance between Yin and Yang is not fixed and can fluctuate based on a variety of variables, including a person's constitution, environment, and lifestyle.

Shiatsu seeks to restore or maintain this equilibrium by working with the body's energy system and enhancing the body's natural healing capabilities.

Yin and Yang is a fundamental principle in shiatsu and TCM, representing forces that are believed to be present in all aspects of the universe, including the human body.

Shiatsu techniques are used to restore or maintain the balance of Yin and Yang by regulating the passage of Qi along the meridians and enhancing the body's natural healing capabilities.

Pressure Techniques: Thumb, Palm, Elbow, And Knee Techniques

Shiatsu employs a variety of pressure techniques to stimulate or numb particular acupressure points along the meridians in order to regulate the passage of Qi and promote healing.

Depending on the recipient's particular needs and preferences, these techniques may entail the use of the thumb, palm, elbow, and knee.

• In shiatsu, the thumb is typically used to administer concentrated pressure to specific acupressure points. The practitioner may exert targeted and controlled pressure using the thumb pad, the point, or the side of the thumb.

Thumb techniques are frequently used for precise, localized pressure on small acupressure points, and the intensity can be adjusted according to the recipient's comfort.

• Palm Techniques: In shiatsu, the palm is used to apply broader, more diffuse pressure to larger body areas. The practitioner may apply pressure using the entire palm or various sections of the palm, such as the heel, the base of the fingers, or the edge.

Palm techniques are frequently applied to larger areas, such as the back or the limbs, and can be performed with sweeping, kneading, or rocking motions to stimulate the passage of Qi and promote relaxation.

• In shiatsu, the elbow is used to apply deeper and more intensive pressure. The practitioner can apply pressure to specific acupressure points or areas of tension using the skeletal portion of the elbow or the soft tissue surrounding it.

It is common to use elbow techniques for deep tissue therapy or to address areas with tight muscles or knots, as they can apply a stronger and more penetrating pressure.

• Knee Techniques: The knee is utilized less frequently in shiatsu, but it can be used for specific techniques that require a greater amount of pressure or leverage.

The practitioner may employ the knee to apply pressure to larger muscles or areas requiring greater intensity, such as the buttocks or the quadriceps. Knee techniques require correct body mechanics and caution to ensure the recipient's safety and comfort.

It is essential to remember that shiatsu pressure techniques should be applied with sensitivity and consideration for the recipient's comfort and tolerance.

The pressure should be firm but not excruciating, and the practitioner should always check with the patient to ensure that it is within their comfort range.

Additionally, the practitioner must maintain appropriate body mechanics and posture to avoid strain or injury.

Shiatsu utilizes a variety of pressure techniques, including thumb, palm, elbow, and knee techniques, to stimulate or sedate specific acupressure points and facilitate the flow of Qi for therapeutic purposes.

Technique selection depends on the recipient's specific requirements and preferences, and safe and effective shiatsu practice requires proper application and communication.

CHAPTER FOUR
Enhancing Flexibility And Movement By Stretching And Joint Mobilization

Stretching and joint mobilization are essential components of Shiatsu that seek to improve the body's flexibility and mobility. These techniques are used to alleviate tension, increase range of motion, and promote relaxation and well-being on a global scale.

• Shiatsu integrates a variety of stretching techniques to aid in the release of muscular, fascial, and connective tissue tension. In Shiatsu, stretching is typically performed slowly and mindfully, with the practitioner tenderly guiding the recipient's body into safe and comfortable stretches.

Stretching can be passive, in which the recipient remains still while the practitioner moves, or active, in which the recipient actively participates in the stretch. Stretching in Shiatsu aims to elongate muscles, increase joint mobility, and induce relaxation.

• Joint Mobilization Joint mobilization is a Shiatsu technique used to increase joint mobility and alleviate joint rigidity. It entails gentle joint movements in various directions, such as rotations, glides, and traction, to restore normal joint function and relieve tension.

Joint mobilization can be performed on various body joints, including the spine, shoulders, hips, knees, and ankles. Generally, the practitioner uses gradual, controlled movements and works within the recipient's comfort level.

Stretching and joint mobilization are performed mindfully and with consideration for the recipient's comfort and limitations in Shiatsu. Throughout the session, the practitioner communicates with the recipient to ensure that the stretches and joint movements are painless and do not cause discomfort. The practitioner must also maintain proper body mechanics and posture to ensure their own safety and prevent strain or injury.

Stretching and joint mobilization in Shiatsu result in increased flexibility, range of motion, decreased muscle tension, enhanced circulation, and enhanced relaxation.

These techniques can be especially advantageous for individuals with musculoskeletal disorders, limited mobility, or muscle and joint tension.

In conclusion, stretching and joint mobilization are essential Shiatsu techniques that enhance the body's flexibility and mobility. These techniques, when executed with awareness, proper communication, and consideration for the recipient's comfort and limitations, can provide numerous benefits for the recipient's health and well-being as a whole.

The Cultivation Of Mindfulness And Relaxation Through Respiration And Meditation In Shiatsu

Breathing and meditation are fundamental components of Shiatsu that emphasize the cultivation of mindfulness and relaxation. They are utilized to enhance the therapeutic effects of Shiatsu by inducing profound relaxation, calming the mind, and fostering the body's natural healing processes.

• Conscious respiration is an essential component of Shiatsu practice. Throughout the session, both the recipient and the practitioner are encouraged to engage in slow, profound, and mindful breathing.

Deep breathing stimulates the parasympathetic nervous system, which promotes relaxation, reduces tension, and supports the body's natural healing processes. It also facilitates a connection between the recipient and the practitioner, resulting in a harmonious and synchronized energy flow throughout the session.

- Shiatsu frequently employs meditation techniques to cultivate mindfulness and promote relaxation. The practitioner may instruct the recipient in various types of meditation, including mindfulness meditation, body scan meditation, and guided imagery.

These techniques aid in calming the mind, enhancing relaxation, and fostering self-awareness. Shiatsu meditation enables the recipient to be more present in the moment, to connect with their body, and to release tension or stress.

In Shiatsu, breathing and meditation create a holistic healing approach that addresses the physical, mental, and emotional aspects of health. They induce a state of profound relaxation, allowing the body to release tension, reduce stress, and activate its natural healing mechanisms.

Shiatsu's combination of breathing and meditation serves to calm the nervous system, balance the body's energy flow, and create an environment conducive to healing.

During a Shiatsu session, practitioners are trained to instruct recipients in appropriate breathing techniques and meditation techniques. In order to cultivate mindfulness and relaxation beyond the Shiatsu session, they may also offer guidance on how to incorporate these practices into the recipient's daily life.

Breathing and meditation are crucial components of Shiatsu that emphasize the cultivation of mindfulness and relaxation. They support the body's natural healing processes, induce profound relaxation, and serve to balance the body's energy flow. Breathing and meditation techniques can enhance the therapeutic effects of Shiatsu and contribute to an individual's overall health and well-being.

CHAPTER FIVE
Shiatsu For Frequent Health Problems

As it addresses the body as a whole and seeks to promote balance, relaxation, and natural healing, shiatsu can be beneficial for a wide variety of common health issues. Here are some examples of how Shiatsu can assist with prevalent health issues:

• Shiatsu is known for its ability to induce deep relaxation and promote a sense of calm, which can aid in reducing tension and anxiety. Shiatsu techniques, such as gentle pressure, stretching, and joint mobilization, can help mitigate the physical and mental symptoms of stress and anxiety by releasing muscle tension, calming the nervous system, and inducing a state of relaxation.

• Shiatsu is beneficial for a variety of musculoskeletal conditions, including back discomfort, neck and shoulder tension, joint stiffness, and muscular imbalances. Shiatsu techniques, such as acupressure, stretching, and joint mobilization, can help to mitigate musculoskeletal pain and discomfort by releasing muscle tension, increasing joint mobility, and promoting muscle relaxation.

• Shiatsu can also assist with digestive health issues. Shiatsu techniques, especially those applied to the abdomen, can stimulate digestion, improve circulation in the digestive organs, and mitigate symptoms including bloating, constipation, and indigestion. Shiatsu may also target digestive-related acupressure points and meridians to promote balance and harmony within the body.

• Shiatsu can be beneficial for individuals with sleep issues such as insomnia or disturbed sleep patterns. Shiatsu's relaxation techniques, such as deep breathing, meditation, and mild pressure on specific acupressure points, can aid in calming the nervous system, reducing tension, and inducing a state of relaxation, all of which can improve the quality and quantity of sleep.

• Shiatsu can aid in the treatment of fatigue and low energy by fostering relaxation, enhancing circulation, and balancing the body's energy flow. Shiatsu techniques, such as acupressure, stretching, and joint mobilization, can help to alleviate fatigue and increase energy by releasing tension, stimulating circulation, and revitalizing the body.

• Emotional Well-Being Shiatsu is recognized for its holistic approach, which includes addressing an individual's emotional well-being.

When combined with deep breathing and meditation, shiatsu techniques can help to soothe the mind, release emotional tension, and promote emotional equilibrium. Additionally, shiatsu may involve working with specific acupressure points and meridians associated with emotional health and well-being.

Shiatsu can be a complementary therapy for a variety of prevalent health issues, but it should not be used as a replacement for professional medical advice or treatment.

Always consult a qualified healthcare professional for any health concerns, and work with a certified Shiatsu practitioner for safe, individualized Shiatsu sessions.

Five-Element Theory: Body Energy Balance For Holistic Healing

The Five-Element Theory is a fundamental concept of traditional Chinese medicine (TCM) that is frequently applied in Shiatsu practice. It is a system for comprehending the relationship between the body's energy and the five natural elements: Wood, Fire, Earth, and Metal.

According to the Five-Element Theory, each element corresponds to particular organs, meridians, emotions, and seasons, and imbalances in these elements can result in discord and health problems.

In Shiatsu, the Five-Element Theory is utilized to identify and balance the energy flow of the body, thereby promoting holistic healing. Here is how the Five-Element Theory applies to Shiatsu:

• Assessing the Five Elements The practitioner may use observation, palpation, and inquiry to determine the state of the client's Five Elements. This may involve evaluating the condition of the client's organs, meridians, emotions, and other physical and energetic components.

• On the basis of the assessment, the practitioner may identify imbalances in the Five Elements of the client. For instance, an imbalance of the Wood element may manifest as tension in the liver and gallbladder meridians, irritability, and frustration. If the Fire element is out of balance, it can manifest as excessive heat or agitation in the heart and small intestine meridians, as well as emotional problems like anxiety or insomnia.

• Using Shiatsu techniques such as acupressure, stretching, joint mobilization, and other bodywork techniques, the practitioner restores the client's Five Elements to a state of equilibrium.

This may include the application of pressure and manipulation techniques on specific acupoints and meridians related to the imbalanced elements, as well as the use of other techniques to promote relaxation, circulation, and energy flow within the body.

• By balancing the Five Elements, Shiatsu seeks to support the body's natural healing processes and promote overall well-being. When the body's energy flow is balanced, it can aid in the treatment of not only physical symptoms, but also emotional, mental, and energetic imbalances, thereby fostering holistic healing on multiple levels.

• In addition to Shiatsu techniques, the practitioner may also provide Five-Element Theory-based lifestyle recommendations to promote the client's health and well-being. Depending on the client's Five-Element imbalances, this may involve dietary recommendations, exercise, self-care practices, and stress management techniques.

Five-Element Theory in Shiatsu is not a diagnostic instrument, and Shiatsu practitioners do not diagnose or treat specific medical conditions. It is a holistic approach that seeks to promote balance and harmony in the energy flow of the body, thereby promoting overall health and well-being. Shiatsu should always be used as a complementary therapy in conjunction with conventional medical care, and it is recommended to work with a qualified and certified Shiatsu practitioner for safe, individualized sessions.

CHAPTER SIX
Addressing Age-Related Health Concerns With Shiatsu

Shiatsu's delicate and non-invasive bodywork techniques can address age-related health concerns and promote overall well-being, making it especially beneficial for seniors. Here are some advantages of Shiatsu for senior citizens:

• Shiatsu can help alleviate the chronic discomfort associated with age-related conditions like arthritis, joint stiffness, and muscle tension. Shiatsu's acupressure techniques can aid in the release of tension and obstructions in the body's energy channels, resulting in pain relief and relaxation.

• Improved blood and lymphatic circulation: Shiatsu techniques, such as acupressure and joint mobilization, can improve blood and lymphatic circulation, which can be beneficial for seniors who may experience decreased circulation due to age-related or health-related factors. Enhanced circulation can promote enhanced tissue oxygenation, enhanced immune function, and general vitality.

• Shiatsu can aid in reducing stress and anxiety, which are prevalent concerns among seniors.

The gentle and calming nature of Shiatsu, when combined with deep breathing and mindfulness techniques, can help seniors achieve a state of relaxation and better manage tension.

• Shiatsu involves stretching and joint mobilization techniques that can aid in the improvement of flexibility, range of motion, and joint mobility.

This can be especially helpful for seniors who may experience decreased flexibility and mobility due to aging or certain health conditions, allowing them to maintain or enhance their physical abilities.

• Shiatsu acknowledges the connection between the body, mind, and emotions and seeks to balance the body's energy flow as a whole. This can aid seniors in coping with emotional issues such as anxiety, depression, and mood swings, thereby fostering their emotional and mental health.

• Shiatsu can assist seniors in relaxing and unwinding, resulting in improved sleep quality. As it enables the body to rest, repair, and rejuvenate, better sleep can have a positive effect on overall health and well-being.

• Shiatsu can be tailored to the specific requirements and conditions of elderly patients. Taking into account any health conditions, medications, or physical limitations, shiatsu practitioners can adapt their techniques and pressure levels to meet the specific requirements of senior citizens.

Shiatsu is a complementary therapy and should not be used as a replacement for conventional medical care for seniors.

Before beginning Shiatsu sessions, it is recommended to consult with a qualified and certified Shiatsu practitioner who has experience working with seniors, and to inform them of any health conditions, medications, or concerns. Shiatsu can be a beneficial addition to a senior's wellness regimen, as it promotes physical, emotional, and mental health.

Shiatsu For Athletic Efficiency

Shiatsu can be utilized as a complementary therapy to support and improve athletic performance. Here are some ways in which Shiatsu can benefit athletes and sports enthusiasts:

• Shiatsu can assist in identifying and treating imbalances in the body's energy flow, which may contribute to musculoskeletal imbalances and increase the risk of injuries.

Regular Shiatsu sessions can aid in relieving muscle tension, enhancing joint mobility, and promoting correct alignment, thereby assisting athletes in preventing injuries and maintaining peak physical condition.

• Shiatsu techniques, such as acupressure, stretching, and joint mobilization, can assist in enhancing muscle function, flexibility, and range of motion. Runners, cyclists, and weightlifters, who require specific muscle groups to be conditioned and perform at their peak, can benefit greatly from this.

• Shiatsu can aid in recuperation from training and competitions by promoting relaxation, reducing muscle soreness, and enhancing circulation. This can help athletes recover more quickly and effectively, enabling them to perform at their peak in future training sessions or competitions.

• Shiatsu can assist athletes in managing the tension, anxiety, and nervousness associated with sports performance. Shiatsu's relaxation and mindfulness techniques can assist athletes in calming their minds, enhancing mental concentration, and enhancing their performance under duress.

• Shiatsu is based on the principles of traditional Chinese medicine, which include the concept of modulating the energy flow of the body for optimal health and performance.

By identifying and correcting imbalances in the body's energy channels, Shiatsu can assist athletes in attaining a state of physical and mental equilibrium, which can contribute to enhanced athletic performance.

• Shiatsu can be tailored to the specific requirements and objectives of athletes. Shiatsu practitioners can modify their techniques and levels of pressure to meet the specific needs of athletes, taking into account their sports activities, training regimen, and physical condition.

• Rehabilitation from sports-related injuries Shiatsu can be used as part of a comprehensive rehabilitation program to support the healing process, reduce pain and inflammation, and promote recovery in the case of sports-related injuries.

Shiatsu techniques can aid in improving circulation, relieving muscle tension, and restoring normal joint mobility, thereby supporting the rehabilitation process and allowing athletes to return to their sport more quickly and safely.

Shiatsu should only be utilized as a complementary therapy, not as a replacement for conventional sports training or medical care.

Before beginning Shiatsu sessions, it is recommended to consult with a qualified and certified Shiatsu practitioner who has experience working with athletes and sports performance, and to inform them of any specific concerns or conditions. Shiatsu can be a beneficial addition to an athlete's comprehensive training and wellness regimen, promoting physical, mental, and emotional health and enhancing athletic performance.

CHAPTER SEVEN
Self-Shiatsu Techniques: Shiatsu Practice For Everyday Maintenance

Additionally, shiatsu can be employed as self-care for daily maintenance and wellness. Here are a few self-Shiatsu techniques you can try:

• Hand and Finger Pressures: You can apply gentle pressure to specific acupressure points on your body using your fingertips, thumbs, or palms. For instance, you can use your thumb or fingertips to apply circular or rocking pressure to meridian points on your hands, arms, legs, and feet. This can assist in stimulating energy flow, releasing tension, and promoting relaxation.

• Stretching and Joint Mobilization: To increase flexibility and mobility, you can extend and mobilize your joints gently. For instance, you can gently extend your neck, shoulders, arms, wrists, fingers, spine, hips, knees, ankles, and toes to alleviate tension, increase blood flow, and promote relaxation.

• Practicing deep breathing and mindfulness techniques can help you relax your body and psyche. You can concentrate on your breath and practice slow, deep inhalation while consciously relaxing various body parts. This can aid in reducing stress, calming the psyche, and promoting relaxation.

• You can give yourself a gentle massage on various areas of your body using your hands, fingers, or other tools such as a foam roller or tennis ball. You can use kneading, caressing, or pressing movements to alleviate tension, enhance circulation, and promote relaxation.

• Energy Balancing: You can practice energy balancing exercises, such as Qi Gong or Tai Chi, which consist of movements and postures designed to balance the body's energy flow. These exercises can help bring yin and yang energies into balance, promote relaxation, and improve overall health.

• Daily Shiatsu Routine: You can establish a daily Shiatsu routine that incorporates a combination of the techniques listed above, based on your individual needs and preferences.

Even if you can only devote a few minutes per day to self-Shiatsu practice, strive to maintain a consistent schedule.

It is essential to pay attention to your body and practice self-Shiatsu with caution and awareness.

Before employing self-Shiatsu techniques, it is recommended to consult with a qualified and certified Shiatsu practitioner or healthcare professional if you have specific health concerns or conditions.

They can offer advice and recommendations based on your specific requirements and ensure that you practice safely and effectively. Self-Shiatsu can be a valuable instrument for daily maintenance and self-care, aiding in relaxation, stress reduction, and the promotion of overall health and well-being.

Shiatsu In Everyday Life: Implementing Shiatsu Principles In Everyday Activities

Shiatsu principles can be implemented in daily life to promote health and well-being. Here are some methods for incorporating Shiatsu into your daily life:

• As you walk, practice mindfulness by being entirely present and aware of your body and surroundings. Focus on your breathing, your posture, and the sensations in your feet and legs. You can also incorporate Shiatsu principles by applying moderate pressure to specific acupressure points on your feet while walking, or by imagining energy flowing through your body with each step.

• Pay attention to your sitting posture throughout the day, regardless of whether you are seated at a desk, in a vehicle, or on a chair at home. Sit with your back straight, your shoulders relaxed, and your heels on the ground. While seated, you can also apply Shiatsu techniques, such as hand or finger pressures, to acupressure points on your hands, arms, or legs to relieve tension and promote relaxation.

• Take short breaks throughout the day to exercise self-Shiatsu techniques, including hand or finger pressures, stretching, and joint mobilization. Even during a busy day, these pauses can help you release tension, reduce stress, and promote relaxation.

• Mindful Eating: To practice mindful eating, be completely present and conscious of your food as you consume it. Chew slowly, appreciate the flavors, and focus on the sensations in your mouth, esophagus, and stomach.

To stimulate digestion and promote relaxation, you can also integrate Shiatsu principles by massaging your abdomen in a clockwise direction with your hands before and after meals.

• Twilight Rituals: Incorporate Shiatsu techniques into your twilight rituals to promote relaxation and prepare your body for sleep.

While lying in bed, you can practice self-Shiatsu techniques, such as hand or finger pressures, stretching, and breathing exercises, to relieve stress, soothe the mind, and promote restful sleep.

• Mindfulness and respiration: Throughout the day, practice mindfulness and deep respiration wherever you are. Take a few moments to pause, breathe deeply into your abdomen, and let go of any physical tension. Visualize energy flowing through your body with each inhalation, and use your breath to cultivate relaxation and equilibrium.

• Create a daily self-Shiatsu routine that incorporates various Shiatsu techniques, such as hand or finger pressures, stretching, joint mobilization, deep breathing, and meditation, in order to promote relaxation and well-being.

You can set aside a few minutes per day to practice these techniques, which are adapted to your specific requirements and preferences.

Incorporating Shiatsu principles into your daily life can help you cultivate mindfulness, relaxation, and equilibrium, and improve your health and well-being as a whole. Remember to listen to your body and practice with care and mindfulness, and if you have specific health concerns or conditions, consult a qualified and certified Shiatsu practitioner or healthcare professional.

CHAPTER EIGHT
Shiatsu Practitioners' Self-Care: Nurturing Your Own Health And Well-Being

As a Shiatsu practitioner, you must prioritize your own health and well-being in order to care for others effectively. Here are some suggestions for self-care for Shiatsu practitioners:

• Regular Self-Shiatsu Practice: Integrate regular self-Shiatsu practice into your regimen to alleviate stress, relax, and balance your own energy. You can use various Shiatsu techniques, including hand or finger pressures, stretching, joint mobilization, and breathing exercises, to address your unique requirements and maintain your health.

• Posture and Body Mechanics: During your Shiatsu sessions, pay close attention to your posture and body mechanics. Maintain an upright posture, employ proper body mechanics, and avoid overexertion and strain.

Rather than relying merely on muscle strength, use your body weight and leverage to apply pressure.

• Rest and Recuperation: Ensure that you get sufficient rest and recuperation time to enable your body to heal and rejuvenate.

Prioritize self-care activities, such as adequate sleep, relaxation techniques, and activities that bring you pleasure and rejuvenation, and avoid overworking or overbooking yourself.

• Personal Stress Management: Employ stress management strategies that work for you, such as mindfulness, deep breathing, meditation, or other relaxation techniques. Find healthy methods to manage your own stress and emotions as a Shiatsu practitioner, as stress can negatively affect your health and well-being.

• Nutrition and Hydration: Maintain a well-balanced, nutritious diet and drink enough water throughout the day. Eating nutritious foods and remaining hydrated can help you maintain your energy, concentration, and general health.

• Engage in regular physical activity to maintain your body's strength, flexibility, and equilibrium. Include activities such as yoga, tai chi, and other forms of exercise that complement your Shiatsu practice and promote your overall health and wellbeing.

• Continuing Education and Professional Support: Remain abreast of the most recent advancements in Shiatsu and continue your professional education to improve your skills and knowledge.

When necessary, seek professional support or supervision and interact with fellow Shiatsu practitioners or other healthcare professionals for collaborative support.

• Boundaries and Self-Care Practices: To avoid exhaustion and maintain a healthy work-life balance, establish healthy boundaries in your practice. Prioritize self-care practices and make room for your own well-being, both within and beyond your Shiatsu practice.

Remember that self-care is an essential component of being a compassionate and effective Shiatsu practitioner, not a selfish act. Taking care of your own health and well-being enables you to provide the best possible care to your clients by allowing you to be present in full capacity. As a Shiatsu practitioner, incorporate self-care practices into your daily regimen and make them a priority in order to maintain your health and well-being.

Shiatsu And Vitamins

Although Shiatsu is predominantly a bodywork therapy that focuses on balancing the body's energy, nutrition can also support an individual's overall health and well-being. Here are some intersections between Shiatsu and nutrition:

• Approach based on meridians: In Shiatsu, the concept of meridians, which are the body's energy channels, is fundamental.

These meridians are associated with various organs and body systems, and imbalances in these meridians can result in a variety of health issues. According to traditional Chinese medicine (TCM), upon which Shiatsu is based, each organ is associated with a particular flavor, and incorporating these flavors into your diet can help you balance the energy of the corresponding meridian.

For instance, acidic foods correspond to the Liver meridian, bitter foods to the Heart meridian, and so on. Dietary variety based on the meridian system can support overall health and well-being.

• Shiatsu practitioners may provide recommendations on specific foods or dietary adjustments to support the healing process for specific health concerns.

If a client presents with digestive issues, inflammation, or hormonal imbalances, for instance, a Shiatsu practitioner may recommend dietary changes to support the body's self-healing mechanisms. These recommendations may include avoiding certain foods that exacerbate the condition, integrating foods with specific nutrients that promote healing, or balancing the consumption of various food groups to improve overall health.

• Shiatsu emphasizes mindfulness and being present in the present moment. This also applies to one's orientation to food and eating.

Mindful eating can enhance digestion and promote well-being on a global scale. It involves focusing on the flavor, texture, and aroma of food, chewing methodically and thoroughly, and being aware of hunger and fullness cues. In addition to fostering a healthy relationship with food and promoting balanced eating habits, mindful eating can also cultivate a healthy relationship with food.

• Hydration: Adequate hydration is necessary for overall health and wellbeing. Shiatsu practitioners may emphasize the importance of hydration and regular water consumption to support the body's energy flow, assist digestion, and preserve optimal organ function.

• Shiatsu is a holistic treatment that takes the individual's unique constitution, health condition, and energy imbalances into account. Similar to nutrition, a personalized approach to diet and nutrition can complement the principles of Shiatsu.

A Shiatsu practitioner may work with a client to determine his or her unique nutritional needs and make recommendations based on those needs.

It is essential to note that Shiatsu practitioners are not nutritionists or dieticians, and their nutritional recommendations should not be viewed as a replacement for professional medical advice.

However, incorporating nutrition and mindful eating into Shiatsu practice can provide clients with additional support on their path to overall health and well-being.

For specific dietary recommendations tailored to an individual's unique requirements and health conditions, it is always best to consult with a qualified nutritionist or healthcare professional.

CHAPTER NINE
Shiatsu And Religiousness

Shiatsu, as a holistic bodywork therapy, can be viewed as having a spiritual connection, despite having no religious or spiritual beliefs associated with it. Here are some examples of how Shiatsu can be linked to spirituality:

• Shiatsu emphasizes mindfulness and presence in the present moment.

During the session, practitioners are trained to be entirely present and attentive to the client's body, energy, and breath.

This profound state of presence can create a meditative and mindful space for both the practitioner and the recipient, enabling a deeper connection with oneself and a sense of spiritual connection.

• Shiatsu is based on the concept of energy, and practitioners strive to balance the flow of energy through the body's energy channels, meridians, and acupressure points. The concept of energy is also central to numerous spiritual practices and worldviews, such as Qi (Chi) in traditional Chinese medicine, Prana in Ayurveda, and Ki in Japanese culture.

Spiritual experiences and beliefs can be associated with an increased awareness and comprehension of the subtle energy body, which can be fostered through Shiatsu practice.

• Shiatsu has its origins in Eastern philosophies that emphasize the interconnectedness of nature and the environment with human health and wellbeing.

Numerous spiritual practices and worldviews emphasize the significance of nature and the environment for spiritual development and awareness. Practicing Shiatsu in nature or incorporating natural elements into the treatment space can enhance the therapy's spiritual aspect.

• Shiatsu promotes inner reflection and self-awareness in both the practitioner and the recipient. Shiatsu can facilitate the recipient's self-awareness and investigation of their physical, emotional, and energetic states through attentive listening and mindful touch.

Spiritual practices that entail introspection, self-inquiry, and self-discovery are associated with this process of inner reflection and self-awareness.

• Shiatsu takes a holistic approach to health and wellness, taking into account the physical, emotional, mental, and energetic aspects of a person.

This holistic approach is consistent with numerous spiritual practices that emphasize the integration of body, mind, and spirit for total well-being.

While Shiatsu can be associated with spirituality, it is essential to note that it is not a religious or spiritual practice in and of itself.

The spiritual aspect of Shiatsu is subjective and may vary depending on the practitioner's and recipient's beliefs and perspectives. Respecting the beliefs and boundaries of both the practitioner and the recipient is always essential in Shiatsu practice.

Professionalism And Ethics In Shiatsu Practice

Integrity and professionalism are essential components of all medical practices, including Shiatsu. Shiatsu practitioners must adhere to an ethical code and maintain a high level of professionalism. Here are some important ethical and professional principles in Shiatsu:

• Practitioners are expected to respect the privacy and confidentiality of their clients. Any information shared by the client during the session should be held in strict confidence and only disclosed with the client's consent or as mandated by law.

• Respect for autonomy and informed consent Practitioners must respect their clients' autonomy and decision-making capacity.

The nature of the Shiatsu treatment, including its benefits, risks, and potential side effects, should be thoroughly explained to clients. Clients should be able to make informed decisions about their treatment and have the option to refuse or end sessions at any time.

• Practitioners should maintain appropriate professional boundaries with clients. This includes maintaining a respectful and non-exploitative relationship, avoiding dual relationships that could compromise the therapeutic relationship, and refraining from any sexual or other inappropriate behavior.

• Competence and continuing education: Practitioners of Shiatsu should maintain a high level of competence by routinely updating their knowledge, skills, and techniques through continuing education and professional development.

Practitioners should limit their services to those within their scope of practice and, when necessary, seek consultation or referral.

• Practitioners should provide Shiatsu services to all individuals without regard to race, ethnicity, religion, gender, sexual orientation, disability, or any other trait. Practitioners must also demonstrate cultural sensitivity and respect for diverse cultural beliefs, practices, and traditions.

• Professional appearance and demeanor: Practitioners must always maintain a professional appearance and conduct. This includes dressing appropriately, maintaining sanitation and hygiene, as well as being punctual and dependable.

• Self-care boundaries: Practitioners must prioritize their own physical, emotional, and mental health. Practitioners should be aware of their own limitations and seek support or supervision when necessary to provide clients with Shiatsu services that are safe and effective.

• Practitioners of Shiatsu should conduct their businesses in an ethical and professional manner. This includes providing explicit and transparent information about fees, policies, and procedures, maintaining accurate records, and abiding by all applicable laws and regulations.

By adhering to these ethical principles and upholding professionalism in their Shiatsu practice, practitioners can create a safe, respectful, and effective therapeutic environment for their clients and uphold the honor of the Shiatsu profession. To provide the best possible care for your clients, you must routinely review and update your knowledge of ethical guidelines and standards of professionalism in your practice.

Conclusion

Shiatsu is a holistic bodywork therapy that incorporates traditional Japanese techniques, Traditional Chinese Medicine principles, and modern anatomy and physiology concepts to promote health and well-being.

It involves applying pressure, stretching, and other techniques to stimulate the meridians and acupressure points of the body, balance Yin and Yang, and promote relaxation, flexibility, and movement.

Shiatsu has numerous health and well-being benefits, such as relieving stress and tension, improving circulation, boosting the immune system, reducing pain and discomfort, promoting relaxation and mindfulness, enhancing flexibility and movement, and promoting overall physical, mental, and emotional health.

Shiatsu can be used to treat common health issues, such as musculoskeletal disorders, stress-related conditions, digestive disorders, and sleep disorders, and it can be adapted for specific populations, such as the elderly, athletes, and those seeking self-care techniques for daily maintenance.

Individuals can attain a balanced and holistic approach to health and wellbeing by incorporating Shiatsu principles into their daily lives and self-care practices. Shiatsu practitioners should adhere to ethical principles and maintain professionalism in their practice, including respecting client confidentiality, obtaining informed consent, maintaining professional boundaries, seeking continuing education, being culturally sensitive, and placing self-care first.

Overall, Shiatsu is a unique and effective method for promoting health and well-being that can be incorporated into a variety of daily activities and practiced with mindfulness and professionalism. It is essential to seek out qualified and trained Shiatsu practitioners for safe and effective treatment, and to always consult a healthcare professional regarding any specific health concerns or conditions.

THE END

www.ingramcontent.com/pod-product-compliance
Lightning Source LLC
Chambersburg PA
CBHW051751250726
48659CB00001B/365